Ideas

—

One of the truly frustrating features of our minds is that the more interesting or pertinent our ideas happen to be, the more they have a tendency to escape our grasp. They streak across consciousness like a comet in the night sky, illuminating everything for an instant, then leaving us back in darkness.

There can be a devilish correlation between how important and necessary a thought is to us and how likely it is to elude our command. The truly precious thoughts have something elusive about them, so inclined are they to simply vanish at the slightest approach of our conscious selves.

A core reason why we can have trouble holding onto our bigger, more essential ideas is because – even though they are frequently crucial to our development – they also tend to induce intense anxiety.

New ideas can threaten the mental status quo and are often sharply at odds with our current commitments and habits. An original thought might, for example, alienate us from what people around us think of as 'normal'. Or it might herald a realisation that we've been pursuing the wrong approach to an important issue in our lives, perhaps for a long time. One part of us may want the comet thought to elude us in order that we won't have to face up to a regret or loss. If we took a given new idea seriously, we might have to abandon a relationship, leave a job, ditch a friend, apologise to someone or break a habit.

To encourage ourselves to know our minds, a blunt demand that we should 'think harder' may not be the best approach. In order to give new, important ideas the best possible chance of developing, we may have to lie in wait for them with some of the patience of an astronomer.

We should accept that our brains are strange, delicate instruments that evade our direct commands and are perplexingly talented at warding off the very ideas that might save us or help us flourish.

To join The School of Life community and find out more,
scan below:

The School of Life publishes a range of books on essential topics in psychological and emotional life, including relationships, parenting, friendship, careers and fulfilment. The aim is always to help us to understand ourselves better and thereby to grow calmer, less confused and more purposeful. Discover our full range of titles, including books for children, here:

www.theschooloflife.com/books

The School of Life also offers a comprehensive therapy service, which complements, and draws upon, our published works:

www.theschooloflife.com/therapy

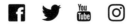